Yoga:
A Man's Guide

The 30 Most Powerful Yoga Poses to
Sharpen Your Mind and Strengthen Your Body in
Just 10 Minutes a Day

Olivia Summers

Published in The USA by:

Success Life Publishing

125 Thomas Burke Dr.

Hillsborough, NC 27278

Copyright © 2015 by Olivia Summers

ISBN-10: 1512243051

Disclaimer

Every effort has been made to accurately represent this book and its potential. Results vary with every individual, and your results may or may not be different from those depicted. No promises, guarantees or warranties, whether stated or implied, have been made that you will produce any specific result from this book. Your efforts are individual and unique, and may vary from those shown. Your success depends on your efforts, background and motivation.

The material in this publication is provided for educational and informational purposes only and is not intended as medical advice. The information contained in this book should not be used to diagnose or treat any illness, metabolic disorder, disease or health problem. Always consult your physician or health care provider before beginning any nutrition or exercise program. Use of the programs, advice, and information contained in this book is at the sole choice and risk of the reader.

Table of Contents

Introduction 1

Tips for Beginners 4

   The Basics.. 4

   Why Yoga *is* For Men... 6

   Health Benefits 7

   To Keep in Mind.. 10

   Modifications 11

Warm-Up Sequences 13

   Sun Salutations... 13

   Sun Salutation A 14

   Sun Salutation B 15

The Poses 19

Day 1: Mountain Pose 20

Day 2: Bird Dog Pose 23

Day 3: Horse Pose..25

Day 4: Cat-Cow Pose 28

Day 5: Forward Fold 30

Day 6: Standing Half Forward Bend 32

Day 7: Plank Pose 34

Day 8: Cobra Pose..35

Day 9: Downward Facing Dog.. 37

Day 10: Low Lunge... 39

Day 11: Half Front Splits 41

Day 12: High Lunge 43

Day 13: Standing Side Stretch... 45

Day 14: Chair Pose... 47

Day 15: Lizard Pose.. 49

Day 16: Warrior I.. 51

Day 17: Warrior II... 53

Day 18: Warrior III.. 55

Day 19: Reverse Warrior 57

Day 20: Extended Triangle Pose... 59

Day 21: Wide-Legged Forward Fold 61

Day 22: Eagle Pose.. 63

Day 23: Kneeling Quad Stretch.. 65

Day 24: Child's Pose... 67

Day 25: Boat Pose... 68

Day 26: Superman Pose.. 70

Day 27: Bridge Pose 71

Day 28: Bow Pose... 73

Day 29: Hero Pose.. 75

Day 30: Reclining Big Toe Poe 77

Create Your Own Workout Routine **79**

Yoga Sequencing 101...79

How To Do It 79

Breathing Techniques **84**

Is it Really That Important?...84

So how do we develop this habit? 85

Here's how to do it…...85

Working Your Core **87**

Creating Abs of Steel...87

How To Do Them...88

Dolphin Plank..88

Side-to-Side Dolphin Plank 88

Dolphin Plank Oblique Variation...89

Three-Legged Downward Dog...91

Knee-to-Arm Plank 91

Knee-to-Arm Chaturanga 92

Arm-Balance Split 93

Handstand 94

Yoga and Your Sex Life **96**

Yoga in the Bedroom 96

The Specifics..97

Yoga for Recovery **100**

Restorative Yoga 100

Conclusion **102**

Introduction

Hey guys! Thanks for purchasing my book "Yoga: A Man's Guide." My name is Olivia Summers and I'm a Certified Yoga Teacher and for the duration of this book I'm going to be your personal yoga coach. Be warned, though: I'm a little bossy. I hope you can handle it! Haha.

Now, one thing you might be asking yourself is: "What do *you* know about teaching yoga to men?" Believe it or not, I get lots of guys in and out of my class room that are eager to learn all different forms of yoga. It is definitely no longer just for women and it actually never has been—that's just a recent belief adopted by Western culture. You gotta love gender stereotypes.

Anyway, in this book I'm going to break down the ins and outs of yoga in easy-to-understand, never-boring language. We're going to cover all the basics and then some so that you can have a solid foundation for whatever direction you'd like to go with your yoga workouts. I'll even give you some tips for creating your own yoga fitness routines.

In this book I use 30 Days as a guideline for getting through the poses. Keep in mind, though it's just a guideline. You can spend as much time as you'd like on each pose; there's no rush.

I suggest spending at least 10 minutes as you're starting point for learning each pose. It's acceptable to learn them in this time frame; however, you will gain a much better perspective of yoga just by committing to that amount of time each day.

However, if you really want to boost your practice and flexibility, I would suggest spending as many days as you'd like on each pose until you feel like you've "got it." For some people this might be a few days, for others it may just be the 10 minutes.

Another suggestion I'd like for you to keep in mind as you move through each pose—or "day"—is that if you really want to cut down on your learning curve and the time it takes you to go from newbie to advanced is to practice each yoga pose that you've learned up until this point.

So for example, if you're on Day 8, start your workout for the day with the poses from Day 1 all the way up until Day 8. This will keep the poses fresh in your mind and also work more parts of your body. Once you get to Day 30 you'll have an entire workout at your disposal.

Again, thank you for purchasing my book and I hope that it helps you to have a better understanding of what yoga is (and what it's *not*) and how it can fit into your life.

Tips for Beginners

Unlike most yoga books we're not going to go over the history of yoga and all its many traditions. I respect the culture of yoga and I think it's important, but for the sake of brevity and simplicity we're going to get right to the heart of things.

If you are interested in learning more about the philosophies of yoga or its history, feel free to check out some of my other books on the subject.

The Basics

There are lots of common misconceptions about yoga— especially when it comes to men practicing it—so let's get those out of the way first.

For starters...*yoga is not a religion or a cult.* Yes, there are plenty of instructors (myself included), that lead chants for spiritual purposes, burn incense or even speak of prana (life force) and chakras (energy centers in the body). But this stuff shouldn't scare you away from practicing yoga!

One of the things that I love about yoga is that it's something different for every single person who practices it—so embrace your version of it. Even if it's nothing more than focusing on your poses and breathing, it's nothing to sweat.

And no...*you don't have to be flexible.* In fact, half the reason to start practicing yoga is to increase your flexibility so it's perfectly okay and normal to not be able to do a super deep lunge or the splits when you first hit the mat. Just remember to take it at your own pace and listen to the signals your body is giving you.

Oh and another thing: *yoga is not girly or easy,* for that matter. A lot of people believe that a yoga session is just a walk in the park and is barely capable of making you break a sweat. If you've ever attempted even the "easiest" of yoga poses, then you know this just isn't true. Yoga is an incredible workout that has the potential to torch upward of 500 calories if you're doing something like Vinyasa Flow or PowerYoga—or even Bikram.

As for yoga being a "girl thing" we'll cover that in the next section.

Why Yoga *is* For Men

So unfortunately we're still dealing with the whole "yoga is for girls" issue. I'm not sure why this ever got started in the first place, considering yoga originated in India over 5,000 years ago thanks to a bunch of *male* gurus.

In fact, one of the most beneficial yogic texts that exists was written by Patanjali—who was, no surprise, a man. So I can assure you, long before yoga pants were popularized and the art of yoga was sexualized...its roots were deeply grounded in masculinity.

So how can yoga *still* be for men, if the majority of yoga classes are overrun by the female population? The answer is simple: it's for *everyone*. And if you don't feel comfortable going to yoga classes that are predominately occupied by females then try taking a Broga class (yoga classes specifically for males) in your area or see if your friends want to start a meet-up yoga group.

I promise, though, it's not nearly as awkward as you think it will be after the first couple times going to a group class. You'll get used to it. Besides, it's not just men that get nervous going to yoga classes—women feel intimidated as well.

Another option is to do your yoga workouts at home. This is personally my favorite way to do yoga, as it's much less distracting and can be personalized exactly to fit your needs and goals.

Which leads me to my next point—the health benefits of yoga!

Health Benefits

The health benefits of yoga are varied and seemingly endless. I'm sure you've heard all about how yoga can reduce stress and increase flexibility...but what else?

Balance— With yoga you'll learn to engage muscles that you aren't used to having to rely on, which will in turn improve your overall stability and balance.

Endurance— By practicing yoga regularly, you'll also increase your performance output in other forms of physical exercise. Whether it's during a heated a game of basketball or in the bedroom you'll have much greater energy levels because of yoga.

Core Strength— The core is the powerhouse of your body and yoga helps teach you how to engage it properly in all aspects of your life. When your core is strong you'll have better posture, which means you can say "Buh-bye!" to back pain.

Mind-Body Control— One of the great benefits of regular yoga practice is that it helps you hone in on your mental distractions and stressors and eventually you learn to ignore them or even let them go altogether. When it comes to your body, you'll be much more aware of each and every part and be able to operate at your optimal level—always.

Improved Strength Overall— By utilizing even the most minute muscles in your body during each pose, you'll be developing incredible strength in areas you never knew existed. I'm not saying yoga will make you ripped, but it will definitely help to tone and shape you into a more streamlined version of yourself.

A Healthier Heart— Since yoga is a major de-stressor, it definitely helps increase the shelf life of your heart and even lower your blood pressure. Not to mention, by reducing the inflammation in your body, you're going to be much less likely to suffer from heart disease. That's reason enough alone to give yoga a chance!

Detoxification— Certain yoga poses and sequences help in the detoxification and cleansing process. How? Well, when it comes to inversions (any pose where your heart is positioned above your head) it helps to keep lymph moving throughout your system and is incredibly efficient at it. Not to mention, the sweating alone is great for purifying your body and skin.

Better Sleep— By reducing stress and helping you achieve a state of inner calm, yoga can actually increase the effectiveness of your sleep. When you practice yoga regularly, your mind becomes clearer and therefore you have an easier time "shutting it off" when you're trying to get to sleep, with less to worry about. I'll take it!

This definitely isn't an exhaustive list of all the amazing health benefits that yoga provides, but I hope that they're compelling enough to convince you to at least give yoga a try if you're still on the fence.

To Keep in Mind

In order to prevent and avoid injury during your yoga workout, there are a few things I want to go over and make you aware of. Yeah, I get that yoga is pretty low-impact and might not seem that intimidating. But that's one of the dangers of it as well. When you jump into the practice without so much as a second thought it opens you up to a lot of subtle (and not-so-subtle) injuries.

Here are a few tips:

- Listen to your body—if something feels painful then you need to pull back. A productive stretch will feel a little bit uncomfortable, but you should still be able to breathe easily and steadily. If you can't, chances are you're too far into it and need to ease up.
- *Always* warm up before going to your static stretches (read: poses)—in the next chapter we'll go over some Sun Salutations—or yoga sequences—that will help get you in the proper state to start your workout.

- Breathing is a major component of a proper and effective yoga workout, so be sure you're checking in with your breathing throughout each pose.
- Be sure to keep a slight bend in your knees so that you aren't overextending your joints and setting yourself up for injury
- Never force your body to do something you think it should be able to do. Just because you were able to do a backbend 15 years ago with no problem doesn't mean you should jump right in and try it today. Give your body time to adjust.

Modifications

Keep in mind that if you suffer from (or simply want to prevent) any form of physical injury—yoga can help! There are plenty of people who have chronic low back pain, sciatica, herniated discs, instability of the knees, muscle cramps, rotator cuff injuries, tendonitis, etc. that have had amazing success and even elimination of these injuries from practicing yoga regularly.

A few months after I first started practicing yoga, I actually got hit by a car while crossing at a crosswalk. Luckily I didn't have any broken bones, but it messed me up pretty badly. I had excruciating neck and back pain (not to mention anxiety) for months and months afterward.

When I finally got up enough motivation to get back in the habit of practicing yoga I was able to eliminate the pain I was experiencing in a matter of a few months *and* get rid of my anxiety surrounding the incident. Needless to say, I'm a firm believer in the amazing healing powers of yoga.

All this is to say that yoga can work for *anyone.* You just have to be committed to it. Yes, there are going to be certain poses that hurt like hell or are basically impossible to get into at first.

The key is to realize that every single pose is modifiable and can be performed to the best of your ability. With consistent practice and discipline you'll get to where you need to be. So don't be afraid to adjust any of the poses in this book or in class to what feels comfortable for you.

Warm-Up Sequences

If you're familiar with any type of workout routine, then you know that warming up is an integral part of it. This is especially true when it comes to static stretching—which is basically what yoga is.

The reason for this is because when you throw your body right into static stretching before your muscles have had a chance to catch up and get pliable, you actually reduce the effectiveness of more dynamic movements and reduce the risk of injury.

Sun Salutations

Yoga's answer to a warm-up sequence comes in the form of various "Sun Salutations"—or in simpler terms: a series of yoga poses that are performed in a flowing, continuous sequence.

When they're done at a brisk pace it can be a great way to get your heart rate up and the sweat flowing. Not to mention, it preps your body for the more gentle, static stretching that will follow. Keep in mind that you should still be able to breathe only through your nose during these movements. If you can't, you're probably pushing yourself too hard.

When it comes to Sun Salutations there are a few different varieties (you can even come up with your own variation once you're more familiar). The main ones are Sun Salutation A, B and C. We'll go over A and B below. If you need guidance with the poses, I've included pictures of the pose sequences.

Sun Salutation A

1) Mountain Pose
2) Upward Salute
3) Standing Forward Fold
4) Half Standing Forward Fold
5) Four-Limbed Staff (Chaturanga)
6) Upward Facing Dog
7) Downward Facing Dog
8) Half Standing Forward Fold
9) Standing Forward Fold
10) Upward Salute
11) Mountain Pose

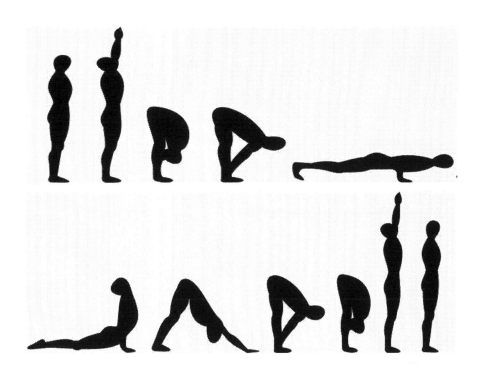

Sun Salutation B

1) Mountain Pose

2) Chair Pose

3) Standing Forward Fold

4) Half Standing Forward Fold

5) Four-Limbed Staff

6) Upward Facing Dog

7) Downward Facing Dog

8) Warrior I (Right Foot)

9) Four-Limbed Staff

10) Upward Facing Dog

11) Downward Facing Dog

12) Warrior I (Left Foot)

13) Four-Limbed Staff

14) Upward Facing Dog

15) Downward Facing Dog

16) Half Standing Forward Fold

17) Standing Forward Fold

18) Chair Pose

19) Mountain Pose

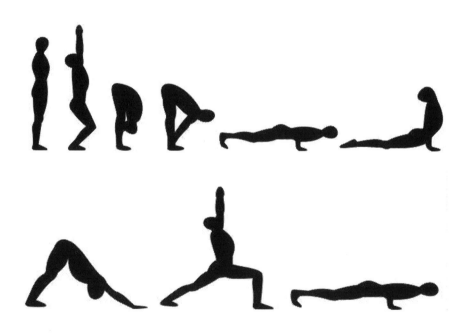

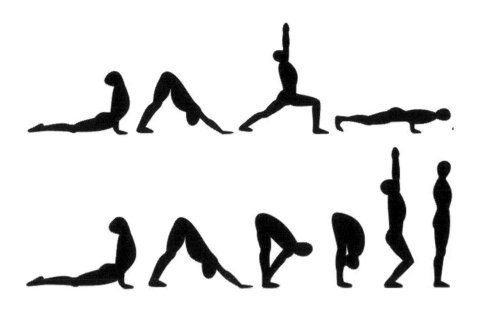

These sequences are great for warming up before your yoga workout, but they're also good for starting your day since they're so invigorating.

Keep in mind that it's advised to do *at least* three rounds of whatever Sun Salutation you choose to warm up with, but preferably more. Once you get conditioned to the poses and feel comfortable you'll increase the number of rounds.

Generally speaking I'll do around 15 before every yoga session. If that seems like it's a bit much, keep in mind that in ancient times they'd do 108 rounds of each Salutation. Yeah, three doesn't seem so bad now, does it?

The Poses

Now for the fun part! Please remember to go at your own pace. If you feel like 10 minutes is enough for you each day—awesome! However, if you prefer to spend more time on each pose I highly recommend it. You'll get much more practice, obviously, and your flexibility will increase at a much faster rate.

As you get comfortable with each pose, try to combine all the poses that you've learned up until the day you are on. For instance, if you're on Day 6: do all poses 1-6 up until the day that you're on so that they stay fresh in your memory and you can build on the flexibility you're developing with each pose.

Above all, just listen to your body and follow its lead and you'll be fine. If something feels wrong, simply don't do it.

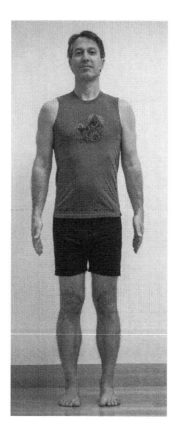

Day 1: Mountain Pose

Step 1: Stand upright so that your big toes are completely flat and touching the floor. Keep your feet about hip width apart and parallel to one another. Now, flex your toes upward and wide—really stretch. This is going to gauge whether or not you're balancing your posture correctly. If you lose balance then most likely you're not centering your weight evenly on all points of your feet so you need to correct your balance so that it's spread evenly on your feet.

Step 2: Contract your thigh muscles and try to lift your kneecaps, but do so without contracting your lower abdomen. Lift the inside of your ankles to help strengthen those inner arches and visualize an imaginary line of energy that spreads the length of your inner thighs to your groin and then from your core (or torso) to your neck, head—all the way out exiting through the crown of your head. Now turn your upper thighs slightly inward and visualize lengthening the tailbone down to the floor while lifting your pubic bone toward your belly button.

Step 3: Now focus on pressing your shoulder blades back and then slowly stretch them out and release down your back. Lift the upper part of your sternum toward the ceiling without pushing the lower part of your ribs outward. Widen and stretch the collarbones, then hang your arms at your sides, palms facing forward.

Step 4: Finally, balance your head completely above the center of your pelvic area. Make sure that your chin is parallel to the floor and keep your mouth and throat soft as well as your eyes.

Stay here and breathe slowly and intentionally for 1 minute or however long you feel comfortable.

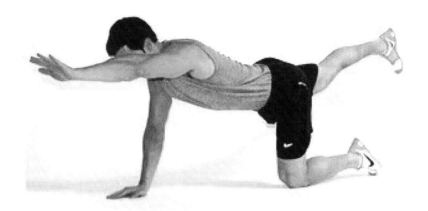

Day 2: Bird Dog Pose

Step 1: Start out on your hands and knees on a yoga mat or soft surface. Be sure to keep your spine and arms in a neutral curve position.

Step 2: Now, slowly extend the right leg backward so that you're in a lunge position—toes turned up and the ball of the foot flat on the floor or mat. The goal here is to keep the pelvis and lower back in a neutral spinal position, never tucking, turning or tipping.

Step 3: From here, if you feel like you're balanced enough, lift the right leg up, parallel to the mat or floor—making sure to not raise it above this height. This will help ensure that the pelvis is aligned correctly.

Step 4: Lastly, extend your opposite arm (left side) forward so that it is also parallel to the mat or floor.

Stay here for up to 16 breaths, then release and repeat on the other side.

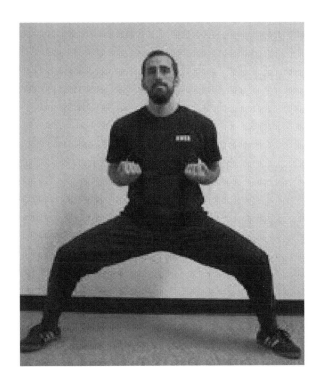

Day 3: Horse Pose

Step 1: Start out at the front of your mat by standing in Mountain Pose, then move your right foot 2 feet or so to the back of the mat with your toes facing out and heels in. Both feet should be at a 45-degree angle.

Step 2: Now, bend deeply with both knees coming out to the sides as you push your hips down into the tops of your knees.

Step 3: Move your arms to shoulder height and also bend the elbows so your fingers are pointing up toward the ceiling. Spread the fingertips apart so that you feel the muscles in your upper back activate as you hold both arms in this position.

Step 4: As you hold here, make sure to keep the core muscles engaged and draw the tailbone toward the mat or floor. Be sure not to hunch over. Keep your torso elongated and all muscles engaged.

Hold here for up to 1 minute.

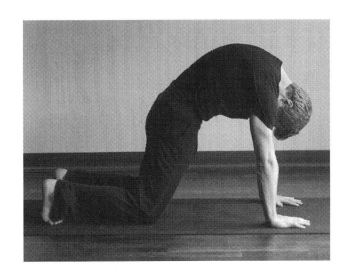

Cat Pose

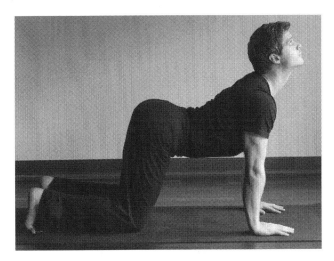

Cow Pose

Day 4: Cat-Cow Pose

Step 1: Start with both hands and knees on the floor. Be sure to keep your knees under the hips and wrists under the shoulders. Your spine should be neutral and back flat. Keep your abdominal muscles engaged and breath in deeply.

Step 2: As you exhale, round the spine upward as far as you can towards the ceiling. It helps if you imagine pulling your belly button into your spine. At the same time pull your chin into your chest and relax your neck. This would be considered the cat pose.

Step 3: When you inhale, arch the back and relax your stomach, keeping everything loose. Raise your head and tailbone upward making sure not to add pressure to your neck. This would be considered the cow pose.

Step 4: Flow back and forth from cat to cow for as long as you like, just be sure to connect the movements with your breathing and really stay conscious of each vertebrae as you inhale and exhale.

Again, you can do this for as long as you wish. It's a great spinal warming exercise and helps alleviate low back pain. I recommend at least 1 minute.

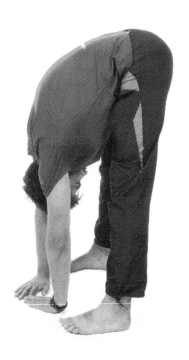

Day 5: Forward Fold

Step 1: Stand in Mountain pose with your hands on your hips. As you exhale, bend slowly forward at your hips. At the same time you should be drawing your stomach inward and engaging your abdominal muscles. You want to focus on lengthening your mid-section as you descend.

Step 2: Now, with your knees as straight as you can keep them, place your fingertips or palms on the floor in front of you. If this is too much of a stretch just grab wherever you can reach to—maybe your ankles or even your calves. Remember not to push yourself too hard.

Step 3: Press your heels into the floor and lift your butt into the air. As you inhale, focus on lengthening your mid-section. As you exhale release yourself deeper into the forward bend.

Step 4: Be mindful of your neck and keep it loose—let it hang freely.

Stay in this pose for 1 minute and then gently bring yourself out of it by unrolling your torso as you inhale.

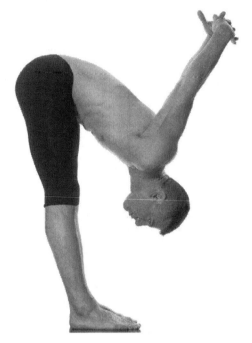

Day 6: Standing Half Forward Bend

Step 1: Start out by bending your head and torso forward toward the floor as close as you can get to your shins. Then from this position, press both palms or your fingertips into the mat beside both feet. If you can't reach this far, it helps to use blocks here.

Step 2: On an inhale, straighten both elbows as you arch your torso back away from the thighs. Concentrate on putting as much length between your pubic bone and belly button as possible.

Step 3: Now, push both palms down into the mat or floor as you pull your sternum up and forward, away from the mat. If you need to you can bend your knees here to help complete this movement, as it will help arch your back.

Step 4: Look straight ahead, being mindful to not cramp your neck up.

Stay here in this position for up to 5 breaths. As you exhale, release and come back up.

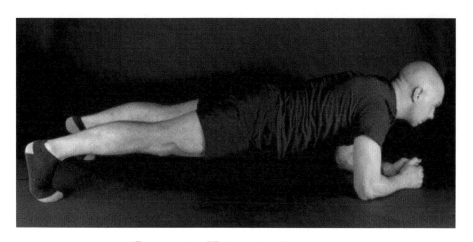

Day 7: Plank Pose

Step 1: Start in Downward Facing Dog. As you inhale bring your torso forward until you have your arms perpendicular to the floor with your shoulders right above your wrists.

Step 2: Be sure to keep your arms straight as you draw your shoulder blades together and broaden your collarbones.

Step 3: Next, engage your core and bring your tailbone toward your heels being sure not to curve your back—you want your spine to be completely straight.

You can stay in this pose for as long as you like or until exhaustion.

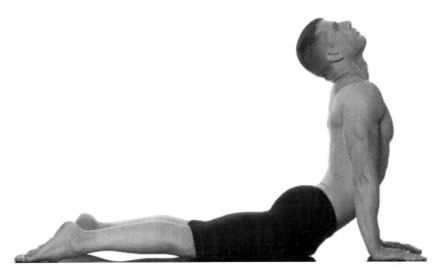

Day 8: Cobra Pose

Step 1: Lie on your stomach in the floor with your legs out behind you and the tops of your feet touching the floor. Next, place your hands on the floor directly under your shoulders as you press your elbows back and into your sides.

Step 2: Place pressure on the tops of your feet and thighs and pubic bone as you press yourself firmly into the floor. As you inhale, straighten your arms and lift your chest off the floor. Make sure that you don't go so far that you're pubic bone is off the floor.

Step 3: Keep your shoulder blades firm as you "puff" your chest forward, lifting through the top of your sternum. Be mindful not to tighten your lower back. If you notice quite a bit of lower back pain or pressure, feel free to widen the distance between your legs as this should help.

Stay in this pose for 30 seconds as you continue to breathe slowly and evenly. On the exhale you can release.

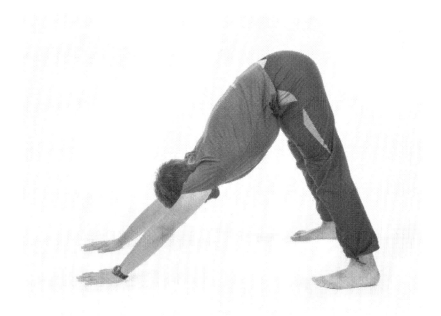

Day 9: Downward Facing Dog

Step 1: Get on the floor on your hands and knees so that your knees are right below the hips and your hands are slightly in front of your shoulders as you keep your toes pointed under.

Step 2: As you exhale, bring your knees away from the mat and keep a slight bend as you lift your heels away from the mat. Focus on lengthening you tailbone and gently press it toward your pubic bone. Lift your butt high toward the ceiling and bring your ankles into the groin.

Step 3: On another exhale stretch your heels down to the mat and straighten your knees—but don't lock them. Keep your arms firm and press your palms into the mat as you draw your shoulder blades back and stretch them. Keep your head in line with your spine making sure to not let it hang.

Stay in this pose for 1 minute.

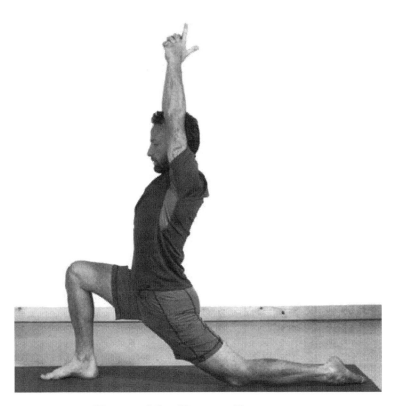

Day 10: Low Lunge

Step 1: Get into Downward Facing Dog. As you exhale bring your right foot up to rest between your hands making sure that the right knee is aligned over the right heel. Next, rest your left knee on the floor and slide it back until you feel a slight stretch in your thigh and groin area. Once you feel the stretch you can rest the top of your left foot on the floor.

Step 2: As you inhale, bring your torso up and in a sweeping motion bring your arms to the sides, perpendicular to the floor. Be sure to keep your chest lifted and your shoulders pressed back.

Step 3: Bring your head up and move your pinkie fingers up to the ceiling. Hold here for a minute and then exhale moving your torso back to your right bringing your hands to the floor and your left toes under. As you exhale again, bring your left knee forward and get back into Downward Facing Dog.

Repeat this pose for the opposite side.

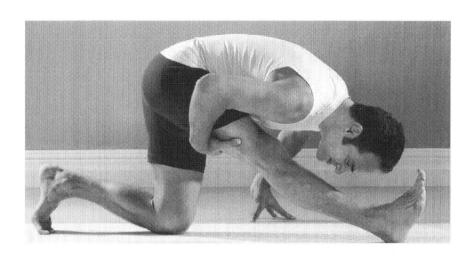

Day 11: Half Front Splits

Step 1: Start off by getting into Downward Facing Dog, then step the right foot to the front between both hands. Be sure to keep a big bend in your front knee as you come into a low lunge position.

Step 2: Now, lower the left knee to the mat so that it's positioned right under your left hip. If you need to, put a folded towel or blanket under this knee if it feels like too much of a stretch. You can also tuck your toes under if you feel unstable here.

Step 3: Next, lift your mid-section up so that it's above your hips and place both hands on your hips while squaring yourself off into the mat. Do this by bringing your left hip forward and right hip backward.

Step 4: From here, straighten your front leg out so that all that's touching the mat is the heel of the right foot and flex it, while keeping a slight bend in the front knee.

Step 5: Next, focus on keep your leg and core muscles engaged as you tilt the pelvic bone forward and fold it over the front leg. Once you've done this, put both hands on two blocks on each side of your front leg—or if you can, on the mat itself.

Step 6: You should pause when there's a good stretch in your front hamstring. Breathe in, here. If you want to increase the stretch a little more you can walk the blocks or your hands forward.

Keep breathing here for up to one minute, then exhale and release. Repeat for the opposite side.

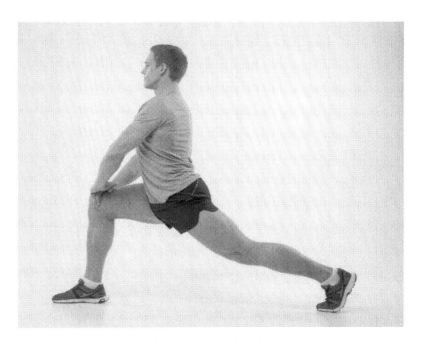

Day 12: High Lunge

Step 1: Position yourself in the Standing Forward Bend pose and bend your knees slightly. As you inhale, step back with your left foot to the edge of your mat, making sure that the ball of the foot is what's on the floor. You want to be back far enough that your right knee forms a right angle.

Step 2: Now, position your torso over your front right thigh and stretch, making yourself as tall as you can. Loosen your groin region by imagining that your right thigh is melting towards the floor while looking forward. At the same time, keep your left thigh firm and pull it up toward the ceiling while you keep your left knee straight and stretch the left heel down toward the floor.

Step 3: As you exhale, step the right foot back and go into Downward Facing Dog. When you inhale again, step your left foot forward between your hands and repeat the lunge on the opposite leg.

Stay in this position for 1 minute, breathing evenly. Then repeat on the opposite side.

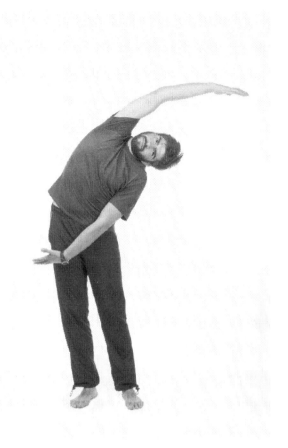

Day 13: Standing Side Stretch

Step 1: Start out in Mountain Pose, then step both feet together so that you're big toes touch and your heels are about a half inch apart.

Step 2: Next, sweep both arms up so that they're positioned above your head. From here you can either put them together in a prayer position or you can clasp your fingers, while pressing the tips of your two pointer fingers together.

Step 3: While in this position take a deep breath inward and then as you exhale, bend to your left.

Step 4: Be sure to keep both feet planted into the mat and the core muscles engaged while breathing into the right side of your body. For more of a challenge you can turn your chest up toward the ceiling as you look upward.

Stay here for a few breaths, then exhale and repeat for the other side.

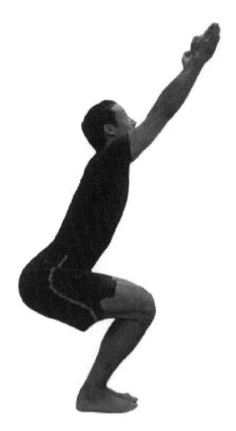

Day 14: Chair Pose

Step 1: Begin in Mountain pose. As you inhale, bring your arms perpendicular to the ground. You can clasp your hands together or you can keep your arms parallel, palms inward—whatever is most comfortable.

Step 2: As you exhale, bend the knees and bring your thighs as parallel to the ground as possible. Your knees will be over your feet and torso will be slightly forward above the thighs until you're at a right angle with the tops of your thighs. Press your thighbones down into your heels.

Step 3: Keep your shoulder blades firm and push your tailbone down toward the ground and inward to your pubic bone. Try to keep your lower back elongated.

Stay in this position for 1 minute. Inhale and lift your arms, as you exhale release and bring your body back into Mountain pose.

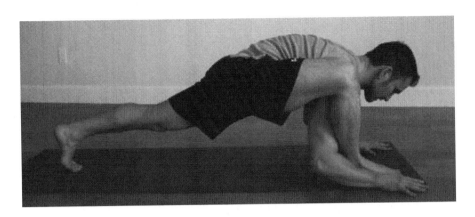

Day 15: Lizard Pose

Step 1: Start by getting into Downward Dog, then bring your right foot up between your hands to the edge of the mat. Your foot should be positioned slightly wider than shoulder-width apart.

Step 2: Relax your hips and let them become heavy. They should naturally settle in a forward and down position. Now, begin walking both hands forward until you can get down on your forearms. If you can't place them flat on the ground be sure to use a block.

Step 3: From here, push your chest out as you lengthen your spine. Keep your chest soft by drawing your shoulder blades inward while straightening the curve of the back.

Step 4: Next, hug your right knee in to your torso so that it's pressing into your inner hip and thigh area of the right leg. If you want to keep your muscles engaged you can keep the left knee lifted off the ground. If that's too much, though, you can lower it to the mat.

Hold this pose for up to 10 breaths, then repeat for the opposite leg.

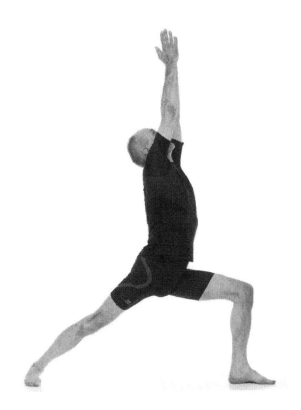

Day 16: Warrior I

Step 1: Start off in Mountain pose and then exhale as you bring your left foot back behind you 3-4 feet. Now, turn your left foot outward to 45 degrees as you keep your right foot forward.

Step 2: Make sure to keep both of your hips facing forward and parallel to the floor as you bring your shoulders forward as well. Inhale and then raise both arms perpendicular to the floor. Be sure to keep them open and shoulder width apart.

Step 3: Reach up towards your fingertips and face your palms inwards while pulling your shoulders back away from your neck. As you exhale engage your ab muscles and bring your pelvic bone down.

Step 4: Carefully move your right knee forward and align the knee over the heel. Keep breathing and make sure the pressure is located in your right heel and not your toes.

Step 5: Be sure to keep your head neutral by either looking forward or by tilting your head back to look up toward your thumbs.

Stay in this pose for up to 1 minute and then repeat on the opposite side.

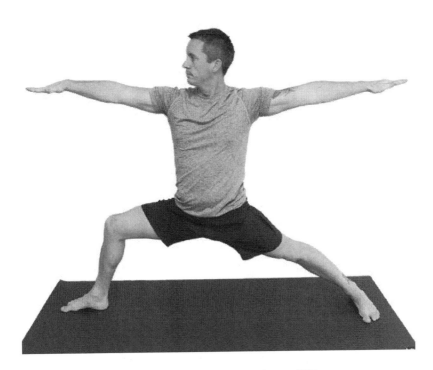

Day 17: Warrior II

Step 1: Start off in Mountain pose and then exhale as you bring your left foot back behind you 3-4 feet. Now, turn your left foot outward to 90 degrees as you move your hips out toward the left and your right knee moves over the center of the right ankle.

Step 2: As you inhale, raise your arms parallel to the floor above your thighs. As you do so keep your shoulder blades wide and open up your chest as you face your palms downward. When you exhale, bend your right knee over your right heel and make sure your balance is evenly dispersed.

Step 3: Tuck your tailbone under and toward the pubic bone. Keep stretching your arms wide and parallel to the ground. Don't lean to your right; keep your sternum tall and neutral.

Step 4: Your eyes should be focused over your right arm to your middle finger.

Stay in this pose for up to 1 minute and then repeat on the opposite side.

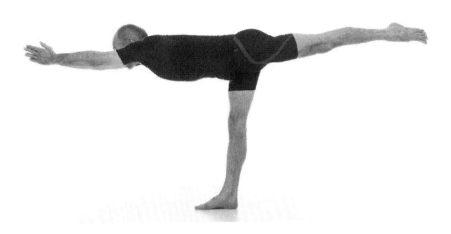

Day 18: Warrior III

Step 1: Start off in Mountain pose and then exhale as you bring your left foot back behind you 2 feet. You should keep your weight focused over your right foot and your toes facing forward.

Step 2: As you move your hands to your hips make sure the hips and shoulders are aligned perpendicular to the floor. Focus on drawing your belly button into your waist, then inhale and bring your left foot off the ground while you lean forward at the hips.

Step 3: Stare straight down as you bend forward from your hips and move yourself parallel to the floor. Be careful not to lock your knees and stop once your hips are aligned.

Step 4: If you want to practice more balance you can stretch your arms out in front of you or to your sides.

Stay in this pose for 5-10 breaths and then repeat for the opposite side.

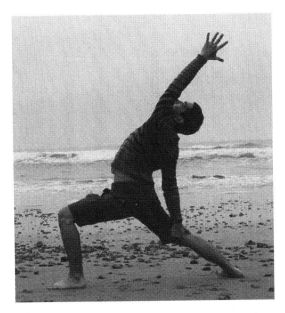

Day 19: Reverse Warrior

To complete this pose, you'll first need to start out in Warrior II. The instructions are as follows.

Step 1: Start off in Mountain pose and then exhale as you bring your left foot back behind you 3-4 feet. Now, turn your left foot outward to 90 degrees as you move your hips out toward the left and your right knee moves over the center of the right ankle.

Step 2: As you inhale, raise your arms parallel to the floor above your thighs. As you do so keep your shoulder blades wide and open up your chest as you face your palms downward. When you exhale, bend your right knee over your right heel and make sure your balance is evenly dispersed.

Step 3: Tuck your tailbone under and toward the pubic bone. Keep stretching your arms wide and parallel to the ground. Don't lean to your right; keep your sternum tall and neutral.

Step 4: Now, bring your back hand down to your back leg with the palm facing downward. Turn your front palm up to the ceiling.

Step 5: As you inhale, reach your front arm up to the ceiling with the palm facing the back of the room. Be mindful to keep the hips open just like in Warrior II, but keep the chest pushed upward to the sky. In this position your neck should be long and neutral and your eyes should be pointing to the sky.

Step 6: Be sure to keep your front knee in a deep bend and the weight evenly distributed on this foot.

Stay in this pose for up to 30 seconds, then repeat for the opposite leg.

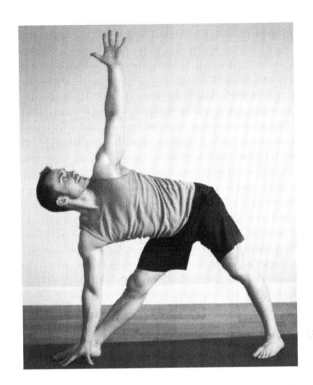

Day 20: Extended Triangle Pose

Step 1: Stand in Mountain pose and as you exhale, spread your legs about 3-4 feet apart. Place your arms in the air parallel to the floor and then reach out to your sides, shoulders wide, palms facing down.

Step 2: Position your left foot slightly to the right and then place your right foot at 90 degrees. Rotate your right thigh so that it's facing outward and the center of your right knee is in line with your ankle.

Step 3: Now, exhale and bend your torso to the right placing it over your right leg. Do not bend at the waist, but rather at your hip. Strengthen your left leg and press your left heel into the floor. Rotate your torso to the left and let your left hip move forward a bit.

Step 4: Next you can rest your right hand however is comfortable—on the floor, your ankle, shin, etc. Now, stretch and raise your left arm up high to the ceiling lining it up with your shoulders. Be sure to keep your head neutral or you can turn to the left to look up at your left thumb.

Stay in this pose for 1 minute and then slowly inhale and come out of it by raising your arm toward the ceiling and pressing your back heel into the floor. Follow the same steps for your opposite side.

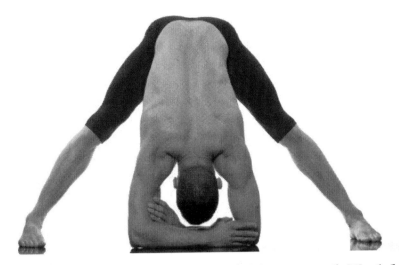

Day 21: Wide-Legged Forward Fold

Step 1: Start off in Mountain pose and face a long edge of your yoga mat. Step your feet apart about 3-4 ½ feet and rest both hands on your hips, making sure your feet are parallel to one another. As you do this, lift the inner arches from your inner ankles as you press outward on the edges of your feet and push each big toe into the floor. Be sure to engage your thigh muscles and then inhale and life the chest so that the front of your torso is longer than the back of your torso.

Step 2: As you exhale, focus on lengthening your mid-section as your lean forward at your hip joints. As your mid-section gets closer to the floor and is almost parallel, push your fingers into the floor so that they're parallel to each other. Position your spine so that it's slightly concave. Then, bring your head up while keeping your neck long and focus your eyes to the ceiling.

Step 3: Be mindful to lengthen your torso by pushing your thighs back and drawing your groin inward to widen your pelvic bone as you breathe here. While maintaining the concave shape of your back and lift of the sternum, move your fingers between both feet. Breathe a few times here and then as you exhale, bend both elbows and lower your mid-section and head into a forward bend. As you move downward, keep as much length as possible in your torso. If you can, rest the top of your head on the mat or floor.

Step 4: Next, push your palms into the floor with your fingers forward. If you're flexible enough to do a full forward bend then you can walk both hands back so that your forearms become perpendicular to the mat and your upper arms are parallel. Be mindful to widen your shoulders across your back and away from your ears.

Breathe here for up to 1 minute.

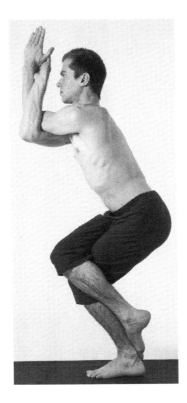

Day 22: Eagle Pose

Step 1: Start out in Mountain pose and then bend your knees a little bit. As you bend your knees, lift the left foot up and balance only on your right foot. Then, cross the left thigh over the right thigh. Be sure to point your left toes down toward the ground, press your foot back and hook the top of your foot behind the bottom part of your right calf. Continue balancing on your right foot.

Step 2: Now, straighten your arms out in front of you, parallel to the ground. Keep your shoulders wide and open then cross your arms in front of your mid-section. Your left arm should be below your right arm as you bend them at the elbows. Your right elbow should be tight against the crook of your left as your raise your forearms so that they're perpendicular to the ground. The backs of the hands should be against each other.

Step 3: Press your right hand to the right and your left hand to the left. Your palms should be facing one another and the thumb of your right hand should be in front of the left pinky finger.

Step 4: Finally, press your palms into each other (as much as you can) and lift the elbows up as your stretch your fingers to the ceiling.

Hold here for 30 seconds or so and then repeat with your arms and legs reversed.

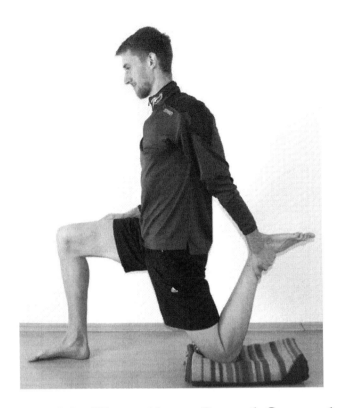

Day 23: Kneeling Quad Stretch

Step 1: Start this pose by getting into Downward Dog, then step the right foot to the front of the mat and put both hands on either side of it onto the mat. You should be in a low lunge position. From here, carefully lower the right knee to the mat.

Step 2: Next, use your right hand to pull your left foot in toward the right hip. Hold it here with your right hand positioned over the top of the left foot, resting the left forearm on the left thigh.

Hold this pose for 5 or so breaths. Then, exhale and release to repeat on the opposite side.

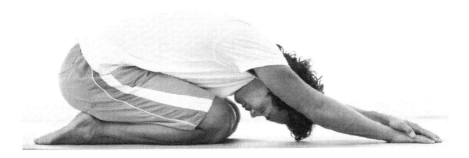

Day 24: Child's Pose

Step 1: Get into a kneeling position on the floor and sit back on your heels. Separate your knees hip width apart.

Step 2: As you exhale, lay your torso down on the mat between your thighs. Once you're settled in, lengthen the tailbone and neck.

Step 3: Now you can position your hands either straight out in front of you, palms toward the ground or you can place them at your sides palms facing up. Whatever is most comfortable to you. After all, this is a resting pose.

Relax in this position for 1 minute or longer, releasing the tension in all areas of your body.

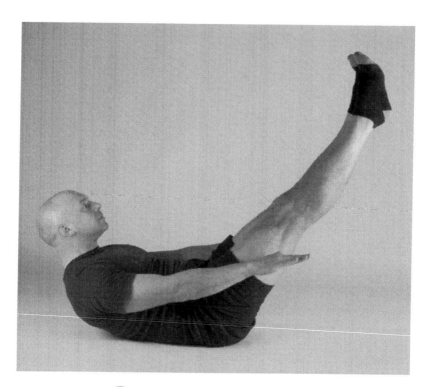

Day 25: Boat Pose

Step 1: In a sitting position put your knees and feet together with your knees bent. Hold the backs of your knees and focus on lengthening the spine as you lean back slightly making sure not to fold over as you find the edge of your butt bones.

Step 2: Stare straight ahead and as you inhale bring your feet a couple inches off the ground, balancing on your butt, breathing in and out as you find your balance.

Step 3: Stay tall as you gently raise your heels to knee level, keeping your knees bent. If you can complete this easily and you're comfortable then let go of your legs and bring your arms forward as you keep chest broad. If you still feel good and steady you can raise your legs at a diagonal in the air in front of you taking care not to round your back.

Stay in this position for as long as you can, but at least 30 seconds.

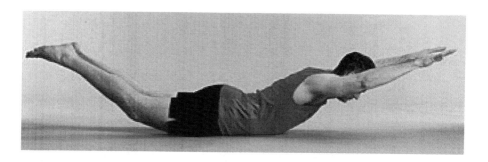

Day 26: Superman Pose

Step 1: Start out by lying on your stomach, toes flat against the mat or floor. Your chin should be resting on the floor.

Step 2: From here, keep both legs together and both feet lightly touching one another. Your arms should be stretched out in front of you as far as you can do it.

Step 3: Then, as you inhale—lift your arms, chest, thighs and legs off of the ground. In this position your arms and legs should not be bent, but rather straight. The focus here should be on lengthening your body from both ends, not on trying to raise up as far as you possibly can.

Breathe here for up to 30 seconds while being mindful of the stretch.

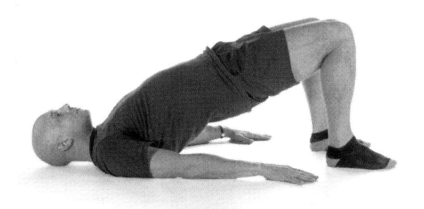

Day 27: Bridge Pose

Step 1: Begin by lying flat on your back. Bring your knees up to a 90-degree angle and place your feet flat on the floor with your heels as close to your glutes as possible.

Step 2: Exhale while pressing your feet and arms firmly into the floor, contract your tailbone up toward your pubic bone and firm your buttocks muscles. Now lift your butt off the floor keeping everything parallel.

Step 3: Place your hands below your back on the floor either flat or you can clasp them together if that's more comfortable.

Keep your abdomen muscles engaged and try to lengthen your back.

Step 4: Keep your chin lifted slightly above your sternum and your shoulder blades firm. To keep your shoulders from closing in, firm your outer arms and broaden the shoulder blades, stretching them across the base of your neck.

Stay in this pose for 1 minute and when you're ready to come out of it, do so by exhaling and rolling each of your vertebrae slowly down onto the floor.

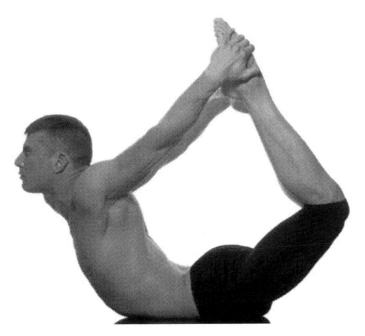

Day 28: Bow Pose

Step 1: Start off lying on your stomach in the floor with your hands on either side of your torso, palms facing up. If you need to, you can roll up a blanket to provide extra cushioning if it hurts your stomach.

Step 2: As you exhale, bend the knees and bring your heels as close to your butt as you can. While doing this, reach back with both hands and grab onto your ankles. Keep your knees hip width apart for the entire length of the pose.

Step 3: On the inhale, lift your heels away from your butt and thighs away from the floor with a significant amount of strength. By doing this you'll pull the upper torso and your head off of the floor. Soften your back muscles and push your tailbone down into the floor. Focus on lifting your thighs and heels higher into the air and press the shoulder blades firmly into your back in order to open up your heart. Be sure to keep the top of your shoulders away from your ears and look straight ahead.

Please note: this pose makes it somewhat difficult to breathe smoothly and deeply, but keep breathing! Focus on breathing into the back of your torso.

Stay in this position for 30 seconds, focusing on your breathing technique. As you exhale, release yourself gently and lie flat for a couple breaths.

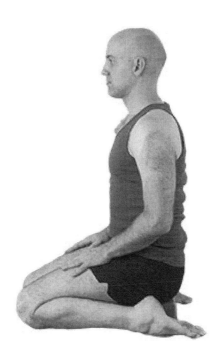

Day 29: Hero Pose

Step 1: Start out by kneeling on your mat with both thighs parallel and making sure your knees are positioned hip width apart.

Step 2: From here, exhale and lean back about halfway, keeping your mid-section tilted forward slightly. Place both thumbs under the backs of your knees and pull your calf muscles down toward your heels. Sit back between your feet.

Step 3: If you can't sit comfortably flat on the floor, then you can raise yourself by placing a telephone book (or other thick book) or block between your feet. Rest both hands in your lap, either palms up or down.

Step 4: Press your shoulder blades into each and lift your chest up and out as you widen your collarbones and focus on lengthening your spine.

Stay in this pose for up to 1 minute.

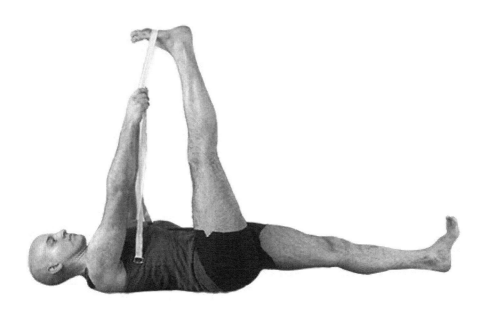

Day 30: Reclining Big Toe Pose

Step 1: Start out by lying on your back on your mat with both legs extended out in front of you. Then, bring your right knee in to your chest so that you can wrap a strap (or article of clothing) around the arch of your foot.

Step 2: Grab it with both of your hands and press your right heel up to the ceiling, extending your leg until it's straight.

Step 3: From here, walk your hands up the strap as high as is comfortable for you. Be focused on keeping your shoulders flat against the mat and widening the collarbone.

Step 4: Your left leg should be engaged and firmly pressed into the mat. Once you're at full extension, press through the ball of both of your big toes.

Breathe here for 30 seconds or so, then exhale and switch to the opposite leg.

Remember: take these poses at your own pace and do what feels right to *your* body. If you need more than 30 days to master these poses, just know that you're not a "failure" or falling behind. Everyone has their own way of learning and for some it may take longer than others—it's normal!

If you get bored with this routine that I've put together for you or you've mastered all the poses and want something that will fit your needs, then keep reading; in the next chapter we'll go over how to put together your own sequence of poses.

Create Your Own Workout Routine

Yoga Sequencing 101

So maybe you've gotten to the point where you feel like you've mastered the sequence that I've designed for you, but maybe you're not quite ready to take a class at a studio.

Don't worry: I've got your back. In this chapter we're going to go over how you can create and develop your own yoga workout sequence that can cater to your personal needs and wants.

How To Do It

Writing up your own yoga workout routine can be both satisfying and also a little nerve-wracking. But nothing beats being able to customize your workout to fit any physical setbacks or personal goals.

A lot of people like to attend yoga classes for the simple reason that they don't know how to practice yoga any other way. Well, today I'm going to empower you to build your own routine and practice your yoga anywhere, anytime—no instructor needed.

Here we go...

Step 1: Take out a piece of paper and a pen and write down all your favorite poses. You don't have to know the proper name or Sanskrit term for each pose—you can identify them in whatever way makes sense to you so that *you* know what the pose is and what benefits it offers. Your list might be very long or quite short. If it's on the short side and you want your routine to be a little longer, you might need to do a little research online or in yoga books or magazines to get ideas for other poses you might be interested in trying.

Step 2: Now, sort each pose into more specific categories—such as inversions, twists, arm balances, forward bends, standing, restoratives or even backbends. If you were so inclined, you could even break it down even further into what each pose targets (legs, arms, core...).

To ensure that you have a balanced routine, you'll want to include poses from each of the categories. Also, don't forget to notate which of your Sun Salutations you're going to do before your workout session.

Step 3: Note that you should start your workout (even before the Sun Salutations) with the Basic Breath Awareness technique. You'll find this in a few pages. This should be done every single time because it's *that* important. With practice, though, you should be able to calm your breathing much faster than you will be able to in the beginning. Just be sure to find a quiet spot where you'll be able to focus on only your breathing for at least five minutes—or however long you feel you need to.

Step 4: One of the most important parts of creating your own workout routine is to decide if you want your workout to be more focused on relaxation, strength-building or energizing (or any combination in between).

Whatever you decide, it's important that the poses you pick match up to your expectations. For instance, if you're going for relaxation then you'll want to choose more calming poses like Child's Pose, Legs-Up-The-Wall—things where you'll be seated or lying down.

If you're going for strength-building then inversions, arm balances or even backbends will fit the bill (think Locust Pose,

Crane Pose, Handstand, etc.).

Lastly, if you're looking to get energized, you'll want to target a more flowing sequence like your Sun Salutations and other poses like the Warrior Poses, Half-Moon Pose, Triangle, etc.

Step 5: This step is the most important step in my book and something you should take to heart. Too many times in my classes I see students fleeing from their mats when we get to this part of our yoga routine, which is unfortunate because it's incredibly beneficial and essential to our overall well-being.

What is it? Well, at the end of every single one of your yoga workouts you should include Savasana—or Corpse Pose. Even if it's not included in the workout!

The reason being, your body and mind need time to adjust to all that has just happened in the last hour or so—we don't want to rush right back to the hustle and bustle of our daily lives before we process and reflect on the journey we've just been on.

By lying on your mat, completely relaxed and at peace,

breathing deeply at the end of each workout you'll be able to experience a rewarding calm that is worth the 5 minutes of delay.

Okay, there you have it! These are the 5 essentials to compiling your very own yoga sequence to fit the needs of your lifestyle.

And who knows, you might get so good at it that you'll decide you want to be a Certified Yoga Teacher so that you can help others find their groove.

Breathing Techniques

Is it Really That Important?

In short: yes! Correct breathing techniques are the foundation of a successful and productive yoga practice. It might sound boring, but it's essential.

Often in yoga classes you'll hear it referred to as 'pranayama' but it's just a fancy way of saying breath work and it's not as intimidating as it might sound. The Sanskrit word 'pranayama' actually translates to "extend the vital life force."

Pretty fitting, right? Breathing is essential to our well-being and livelihood. We can go weeks without food, days without water, but only a few *minutes* without oxygen. So naturally, breathing is something we should pay attention to.

For some reason, though we tend to overlook it and take each breath for granted. With yoga, we're forced to consciously engage with each breath and realize its importance.

So how do we develop this habit?

There are several ways, but one of the most common practices of diaphragmatic breathing is called Basic Breath Awareness.

When you practice this technique you'll learn to breathe more consciously and fully, while at the same time calming your nervous system, reducing anxiety and stress and increasing your self-awareness.

The best part is that you don't have to be mid-Downward Dog to do it. It's accessible anytime.

Here's how to do it...

1) Start by lying on your back, knees bent with your feet flat on the floor (hip-width apart)

2) Place one of your palms on your stomach and just breathe normally for a couple minutes. Do you notice the pattern of your breathing? Is it shallow? Uneven? Labored? Don't judge, just observe.

3) Now, slowly start to relax your breathing—making it as even and smooth as possible. With each breath in, pause briefly before exhaling and likewise after exhaling, pause before breathing in again.

4) Once you've gotten comfortable with this pattern of

breathing, try to concentrate on your abdomen expanding and contracting with each breath. Be mindful to expand it as you inhale and contract it as you exhale—this is what a true, full breath feels like!

Repeat this technique for 10-15 breaths.

Although there are numerous other breathing techniques for meditation and mindfulness purposes, Basic Breath Awareness is one of the easiest and most accessible to start with.

Not only is it a great addition to your workout routine (at the beginning and the end, especially), but you can also utilize it virtually anywhere or anytime that you're feeling stressed or anxious. It even helps if you can't get to sleep—just do a few Basic Breath Awareness repetitions and you'll be dreaming in no time.

Working Your Core

Creating Abs of Steel

Many of the poses in your yoga workout can also double as ab exercises, since so many of them utilize your core muscles. However, there are some specific poses that target your core more than others.

If you're interested in working your abdominal muscles more specifically then the following poses will help with that. All of these should be done to exhaustion—so hold them for as long as possible to really get your abdominals in shape.

Dolphin Plank
Side-to-Side Dolphin Plank
Dolphin Plank Oblique Variation
Three-Legged Downward Dog
Knee-to-Arm Plank
Knee-to-Arm Chaturanga
Arm-Balance Split
Handstand

How To Do Them

Dolphin Plank

Step 1: Start out on your hands and knees, then place the forearms and both palms flat on your mat. Be sure that both elbows are directly below the shoulders and the upper parts of your arms are vertical.

Step 2: Now, slowly walk your feet backward while keeping both your legs and your pelvis lined up with the shoulders. Focus on gently drawing the front of your ribs and lower stomach in toward the spine.

Step 3: Ground your toes into the mat and reach through your pelvis and thighs from your heels. Focus on lifting the back of your head so that you keep the curve of the neck neutral.

Side-to-Side Dolphin Plank

Step 1: Start out on your hands and knees, then place the forearms and both palms flat on your mat. Be sure that both elbows are directly below the shoulders and the upper part of your arms are vertical.

Step 2: Now, slowly walk your feet backward while keeping both your legs and your pelvis lined up with the shoulders. Focus on gently drawing the front of your ribs and lower stomach in toward the spine.

Step 3: Ground your toes into the mat and reach through your pelvis and thighs from your heels. Focus on lifting the back of your head so that you keep the curve of the neck neutral.

Step 4: Now, walk both of your feet to the left, pressing firmly into your right forearm. Then, lift both sides of the pelvis, reaching back through the heels and thighs while focusing on lengthening your body through the top of the head.

Dolphin Plank Oblique Variation

Step 1: Start out on your hands and knees, then place the forearms and both palms flat on your mat. Be sure that both elbows are directly below the shoulders and the upper part of your arms are vertical.

Step 2: Now, slowly walk your feet backward while keeping both your legs and your pelvis lined up with the shoulders. Focus on gently drawing the front of your ribs and lower stomach in toward the spine.

Step 3: Ground your toes into the mat and reach through your pelvis and thighs from your heels. Focus on lifting the back of your head so that you keep the curve of the neck neutral.

Step 4: Next, while keeping both of your forearms flat on the mat, rotate onto the side of your left foot. Stack both feet and legs on top of one another so that they're lined up between your arms.

Step 5: Be sure to distribute your weight on both forearms evenly as you reach down through both feet, lengthening your body through the top of the head. Focus on drawing the lower part of your stomach inward, while reaching your pelvis to your heels.

Three-Legged Downward Dog

Step 1: Start in Downward Dog, then bring the right knee up into the rib cage while simultaneously keeping both hips elevated. If you need to you can lift the left heel off the mat to help you.

Step 2: Now, as you keep your knee by your ribs, push both hands forward while at the same time lifting the pelvis up and pushing down through the left heel. Pause here to engage your core.

Step 3: Lastly, slowly lift the right leg up and back into the air. Hold here to exhaustion, then repeat with the opposite leg.

Knee-to-Arm Plank

Step 1: Start off in Dolphin Plank, then bring your right knee out to your upper right arm. Focus on pressing your knee in to your mid-section. Pause here.

Step 2: Now, slightly lift the front part of your body to the back part of your body, pressing down through the left hell. Focus on pressing your arms in towards each other, but be sure to keep both of them straight.

Step 3: Lengthen your body through the top of your head as you control your breathing. Stay here until exhaustion, then repeat on the opposite side.

Knee-to-Arm Chaturanga

Step 1: Start off in Dolphin Plank, then bring your right knee out to your upper right arm. Focus on pressing your knee in to your mid-section. Pause here.

Step 2: Now, slightly lift the front part of your body to the back part of your body, pressing down through the left hell. Focus on pressing your arms in towards each other, but be sure to keep both of them straight.

Step 3: Lengthen your body through the top of your head as you control your breathing. From here, you're going to bend both elbows so that you're now lowered into the Chaturanga position.

Step 4: Breathe here for up to 5 breaths or until exhaustion, then release and repeat with the other leg.

Arm-Balance Split

Step 1: Start off in Dolphin Plank, then bring your right knee out to your upper right arm. Focus on pressing your knee in to your mid-section. Pause here.

Step 2: Now, slightly lift the front part of your body to the back part of your body, pressing down through the left hell. Focus on pressing your arms in towards each other, but be sure to keep both of them straight.

Step 3: Lengthen your body through the top of your head as you control your breathing. From here, you're going to bend both elbows so that you're now lowered into the Chaturanga position.

Step 4: Finally, lean your chest forward and extend the right leg out to the side until it's straight. Be sure to keep the core muscles engaged and focus on lengthening your back leg. Hold here for as long as you can, then repeat on the other side.

Handstand

Step 1: Start in Downward Facing Dog so that your fingers are a couple of inches away from a wall—shoulder width apart. If you feel like you have tight shoulders you can turn the index fingers out a little, otherwise keep them parallel. Tighten your shoulder blades into your back and pull them to your tailbone while rotating the upper arms out to broaden your shoulder blades. Keep the palms spread and press your index fingers firmly into the floor.

Step 2: Bend one of your knees and step your foot in closer to the wall, while you keep the other one extended through your heel. Get into your pose mindset by doing a few small hops before completely putting yourself upside down. When you're ready, take your extended leg and kick off the floor while at the same time pushing through your other heel to straighten the knee. Once both legs are off the ground, keep your core engaged to help bring your hips over the shoulders. These practice "hops" might be all you can do for now and that's okay—just keep practicing until you feel comfortable and do strengthening poses like Plank to engage your core muscles.

Step 3: However, if you feel strong then go for it. Kick your leg off the ground so that you can bring both legs up onto the wall. If you feel like your groin and armpit areas are tense then the lower back might have a rather deep arch. If you need to lengthen it, draw your ribs into the torso and push your tailbone to your heels while sliding them higher up the wall. Keep your head between your shoulder blades and look out into the center of the room.

Hold here for as long as you can. Having to keep your core muscles engaged really helps to strengthen the lower back as well.

If you practice these eight core-focused yoga poses regularly, you'll start to gain incredible amounts of strength in the powerhouse center of your body. At first, they'll probably feel quite hard to hold—you might max out at 20 seconds.

However, if you're consistent with your workouts you'll start to notice that you're able to hold them for much longer without feeling fatigued—and that's a great feeling!

Yoga and Your Sex Life

Yoga in the Bedroom

Finally, we're to the good stuff! Okay, I'm kidding...well, not really. Obviously, sex has the potential to bring lots of joy and fulfillment into our lives. But what happens if it's less-than-stellar?

Well, believe it or not, yoga has the power to invoke major changes in your sex life—for the better, thankfully.

So what are we talking about here? Tantric sex? Multiple orgasms? Maybe, but not exactly. The benefits that you gain in the bedroom from practicing yoga regularly aren't as they are depicted in pop culture or as mind-blowing as the stories people tell make up.

But just because the benefits that yoga can bring to your sex life aren't what they're advertised to be doesn't mean they don't have incredible merit.

The Specifics

You're more flexible.

This one is basically a "duh!" But it has to be said, right? Obviously yoga improves your flexibility, which means all those crazy bendy positions that you've always wanted to try, are suddenly more accessible.

You become more self-confident.

When you practice yoga regularly, you are forced to take a good, long hard look at yourself. If you don't like what you see it gives you an opportunity to change it. Not to mention, when you're able to see all the amazing feats of strength your body is capable of it's a major confidence booster—like, "Yeah, I did that!" And feelings like that tend to carry over into the bedroom.

You become more present and in-the-moment.

When yoga is part of your workout routine you learn to be more present and mindful of what is occurring in the here and now. In the bedroom this translates to you being able to clear all the clutter in your mind and focus only on the sex that's happening right here and now. Your partner will thank you for this one!

You tend to be more honest and "real."
Oftentimes in relationships we have a tendency to hide our needs and feelings from the other person—whether it's out of fear of rejection or simply of being judged. Yoga helps us deal with these feelings and teaches us to be more open and honest. So, in other words, you won't have a problem letting your needs be heard or expressing what's not working (in a nice way).

You're stronger.
Well, this one is just a plus all-around, right? But in the bedroom it's even better. Sort of along the same lines as the flexibility benefit, you'll now be able to perform more moves that before might have been too difficult to do. Think, movie scenes where men are effortlessly lifting their partners up against the wall and going at it without so much as a second thought. If that wasn't feasible before, give it a few months and check back in—you might be surprised that you can now do things you used to have a hard time doing.

You have more energy and endurance.

Everyone wants to be able to last longer and have more energy. Especially in the bedroom! Because, let's face it: it's not attractive when we're panting and sweating and your partner's in the zone and getting close to climaxing, but then you just can't muster up the energy to keep going. Yeah, that sucks. With yoga as a part of your workout routine you'll be like the Energizer Bunny—trust me, if she doesn't practice yoga then you'll probably be the one wearing her out.

Partner yoga.

Yoga is an amazing way to connect with your partner on a much deeper and intimate level—without ever even having to have sex. Your bond will be strengthened in a way you didn't know was possible. Plus, I mean there's just something about breathing and working together in such close vicinity that is incredibly hot. And working out together is an awesome way to support one another and keep each other accountable.

Yoga for Recovery

As with any type of athletic or physical activity, there is a definite need for recovery for overworked muscles, joints, ligaments and tendons.

Now, it might be true that yoga isn't as "physically demanding" as, say football. However, you work the same parts of your body and strain your muscles in different ways that can still cause injury and problems if you don't respect your body's need for rest and recuperation.

But the good thing about yoga, is that you don't have to take a day off: there are actually specific forms of yoga dedicated to releasing tension and tightness in your muscles that are the result of overexertion. Whether it's from a physically demanding job, pushing yourself to the limit in a certain sport, or even other practices of yoga (like Vinyasa Flow or PowerYoga).

Restorative Yoga

If you're in need of some restorative yoga, then I advise you to attend a class—especially the first few times you practice it.

Why? Because that way you're learning the poses in the proper manner (we don't need any more injuries!) and you can get the full experience.

One of the best parts about restorative yoga is that it's basically naptime for adults. Your teacher will guide you through each relaxing pose and help to clear your mind from the stress and daily distractions we all go through. It's a lot easier to accomplish when you have someone else doing the "thinking" for you and steering your thoughts in the right direction.

In fact, once you've practiced restorative yoga in a class setting, I doubt you'll want to experience it any other way.

Conclusion

Congratulations for sticking it out until the end! You are now educated on all the most important aspects of yoga for men—from why you should do it, to creating your own workout sequence and even how to use yoga as a recovery aide.

Have you completed the full 30 days of yoga poses, yet? If so, how does it feel? I'll bet if you stuck it out for the whole program you're feeling much better when it comes to your flexibility and overall strength and reaping other benefits in your everyday life as well.

You should feel proud of yourself for making it through—even if that doesn't mean you've "completed" all the poses in the book.

But I hope that even if you haven't necessarily finished the 30 Day Challenge, you at least keep pushing yourself each day to become better and stronger than before.

You're never a failure until you stop trying. So remember to never give up. Thanks for Reading!

Made in the USA
Middletown, DE
01 December 2015